SOME THINGS MY FRIENDS SHOULD KNOW ABOUT COVID - 19

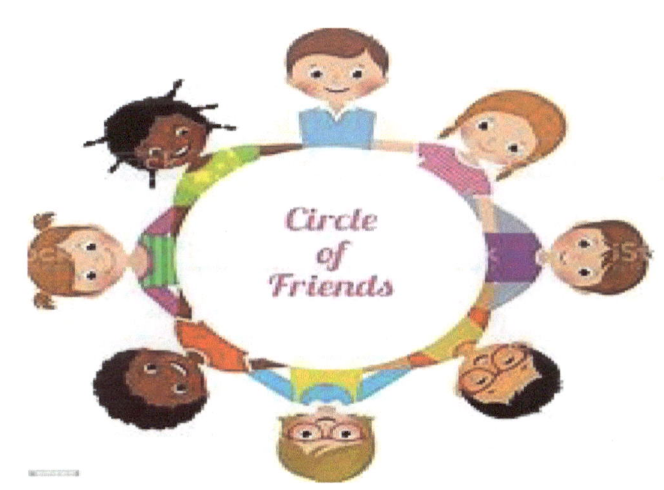

BY DR. ANTHONY T. CRAFT

Published by:
Kindle Direct Publishing

Some Things my Friends Should Know about Covid – 19

Acknowledgements

This Book is dedicated to the memory of my mother, Sadie Mae (Dawkins) Craft April 20, 1936 – July 16, 2016, and to my wife, Janice (Mosley) Craft, who became my better half in matrimony on February 16, 2019.

Some Things my Friends Should Know about Covid-19

Forward

Hello and thank-you for the purchase of my book. I thank GOD for giving me the drive and the ability to formulate the thoughts in my mind and place them into words in the form of this book about our most valuable and protected citizens – our children. I hope that my book adds to your reading enjoyment, knowledge, and awareness. I ask that you stay tuned for many more stories to come.

Some Things my Friends Should Know about Covid-19

Introduction

Thank you for taking the time to purchase and read my book, <u>Some Things my Friends Should Know about Covid – 19</u>. You should want to know that this book should be made absolutely necessary for reading by our children. The children of this world today should be our primary focus and our concentration should be on them. Ultimately, I would like to see this book used by households throughout the world, as this Covid – 19 virus is taking over our free society one virus at a time.

Some Things my Friends Should Know about Covid – 19

Initially, the word was that this virus does not affect children, but different variants of this intense virus has been turning the world upside down. Along with Some Things My Friends Should Know about Covid-19 utilizing everyday safety precautions, the only way to deal with the whole thing is to educate ourselves about the facts. I took the time to base this book solely on my research and daily experience with tuning in to the World Health Organization (WHO), and the Cable News Network (CNN) daily broadcasts about this highly-infectious virus.

I offer this book to children of all ages who can read and comprehend the words. I want children of all ages to be educated enough to the point where they can care for themselves even in the most insignificant manner. This book is filled with facts, information, suggestions, and scientific remedies to help us to survive these circumstances until a solution has been uncovered. Let us come together as a nation and place all concentration on our future – our children.

Chapter 1

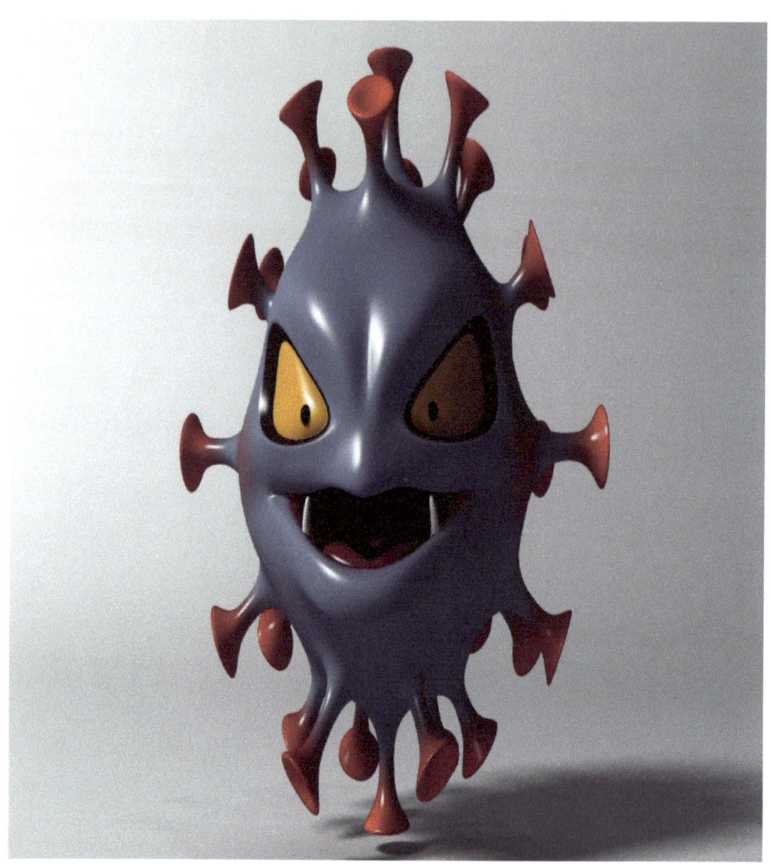

CORONA VIRUS IS AN INFECTION THAT AFFECTS ANIMALS AND ARE PASSED ON TO HUMANS.

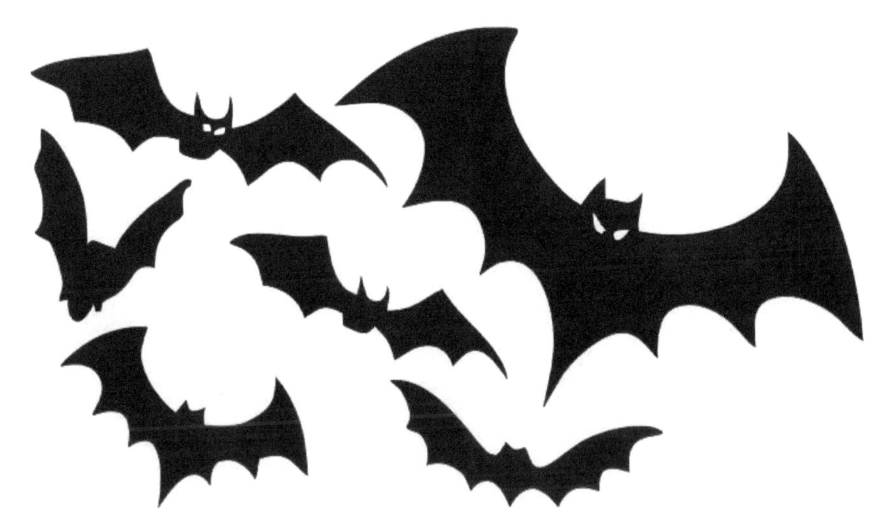

IT IS THOUGHT THAT THE NEW VIRUS, COVID 19 COULD HAVE ORIGINATED IN BATS.

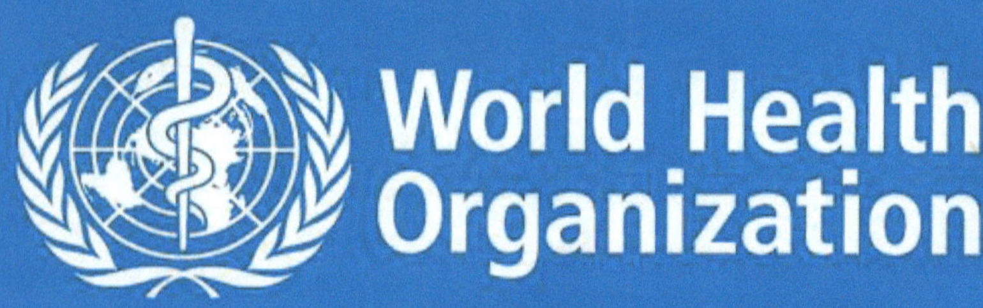

THE WORLD HEALTH ORGANIZATION REPORTS SAY THE COVID-19 VIRUS MOST LIKELY JUMPED FROM ANIMALS TO HUMANS.

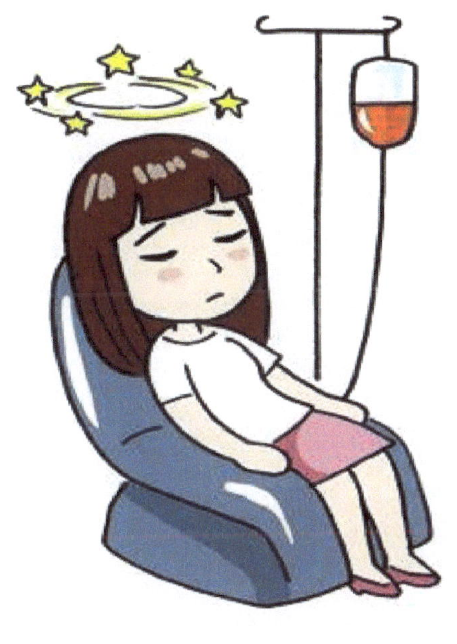

PATIENT ZERO WAS APPARENTLY INFECTED IN WUHAN, CHINA IN OCTOBER OR NOVEMBER OF 2019.

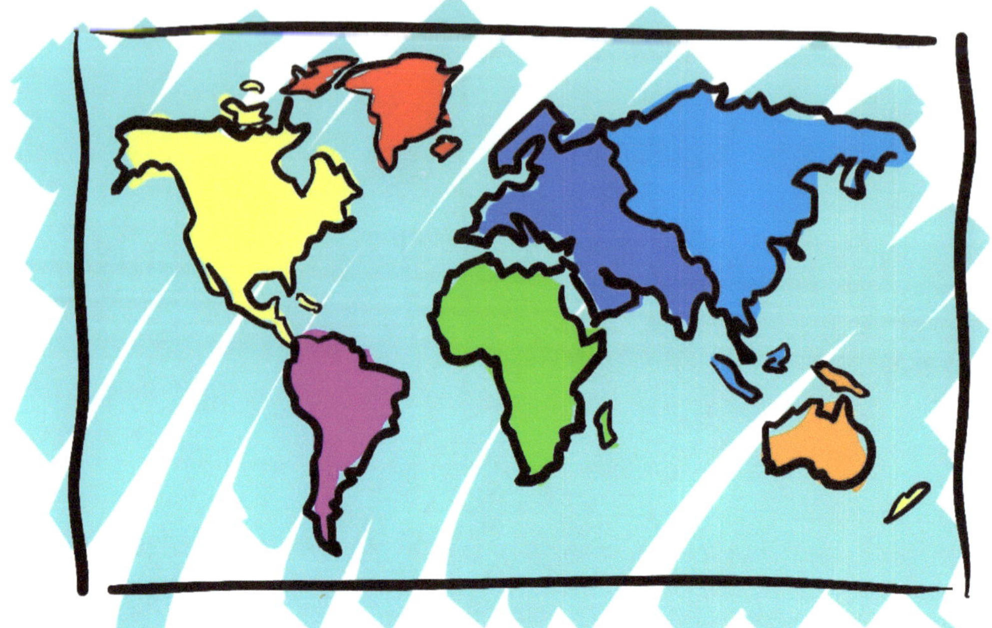

IN DECEMBER OF 2019, THE

CHINESE AUTHORITIES

REPORTED TO THE WORLD THAT

A VIRUS WAS SPREADING.

COVID 19 CASES BEGIN TO

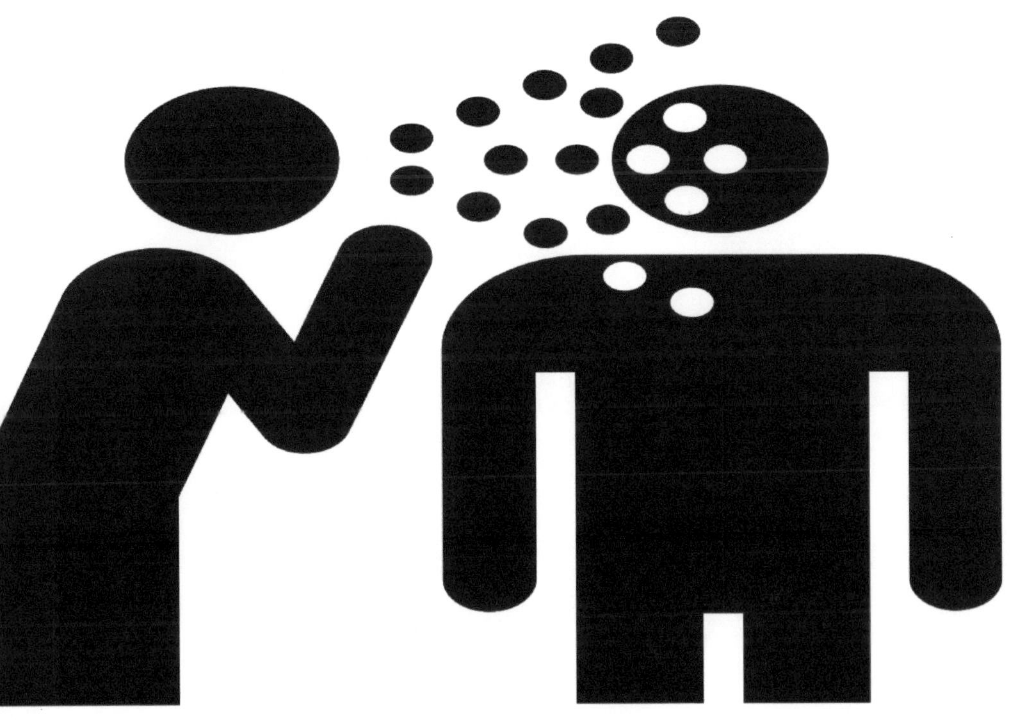

SPREAD WITHIN DAYS.

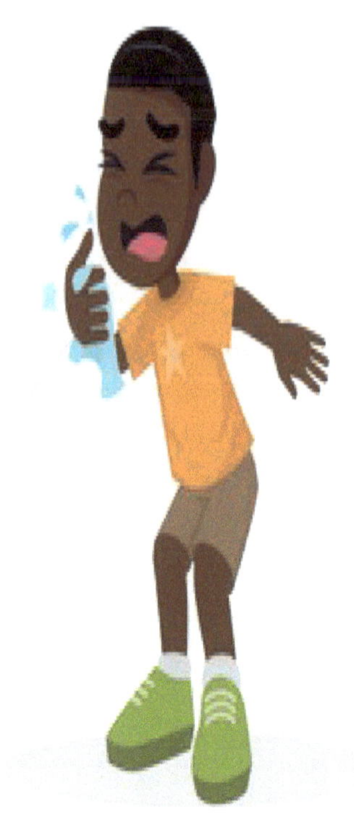

THIS VIRUS CAN ONLY MAKE MORE OF ITSELF BY ENTERING LIVING CELLS (GERMS).

• THROUGH TOUCHING

SURFACES

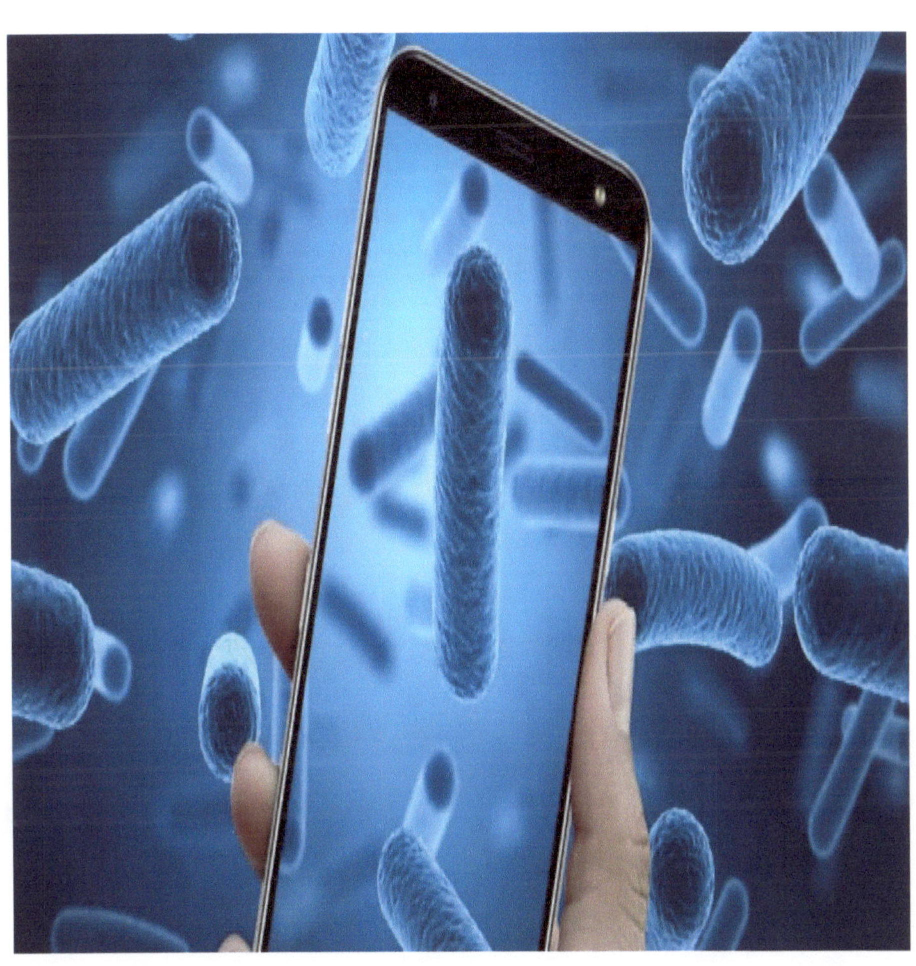

THROUGH DROPLET INFECTION WHEN

COUGHING

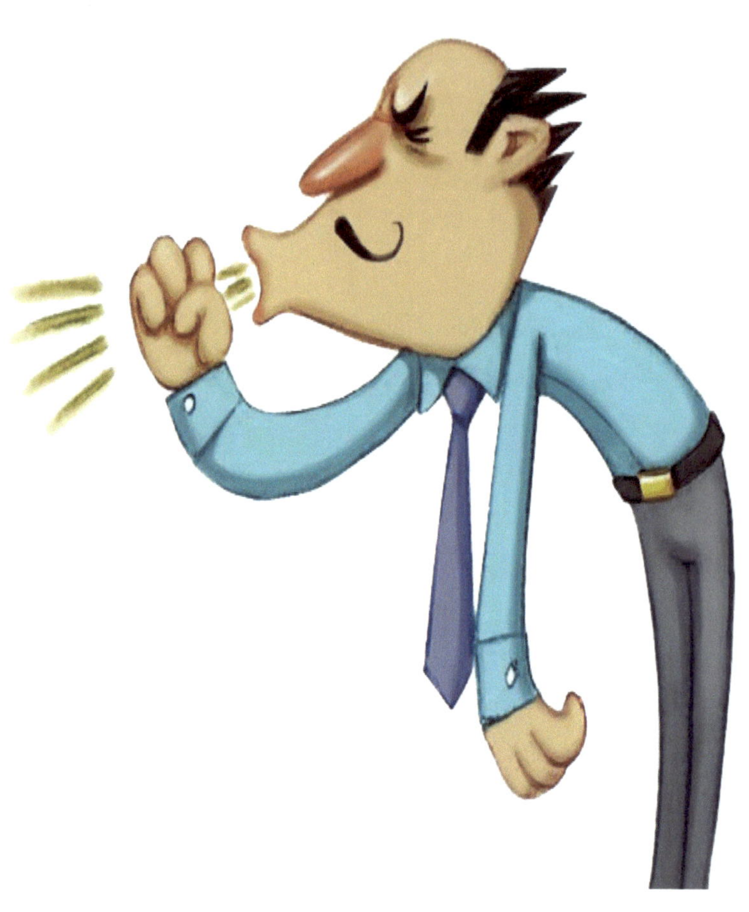

THROUGH TOUCHING

SOMEONE OR SOMETHING

THAT IS INFECTED, THEN

RUBBING YOUR FACE,

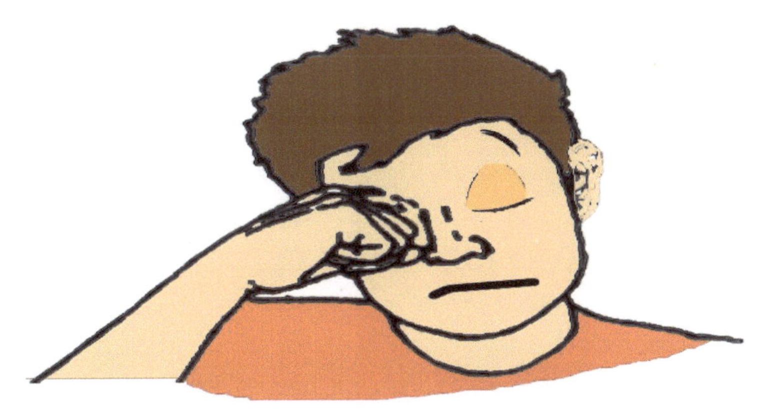

EYES OR NOSE.

COVID 19 VIRUS AFFECTS

LUNGS AND INTESTINES

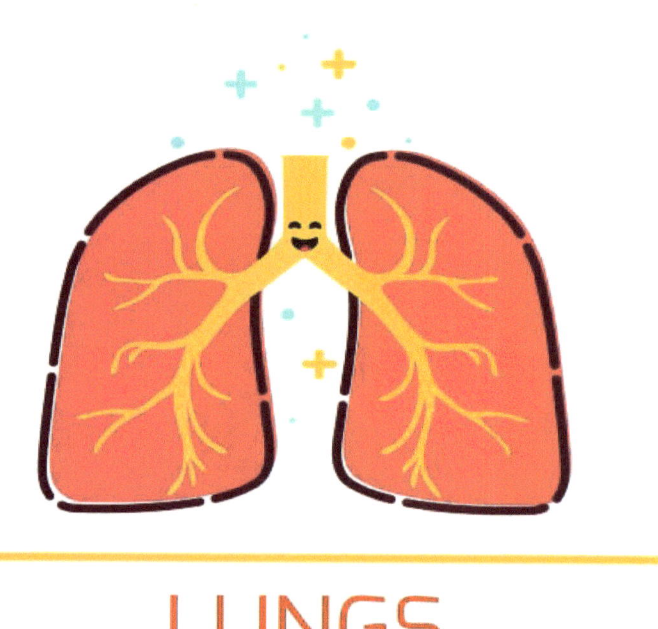

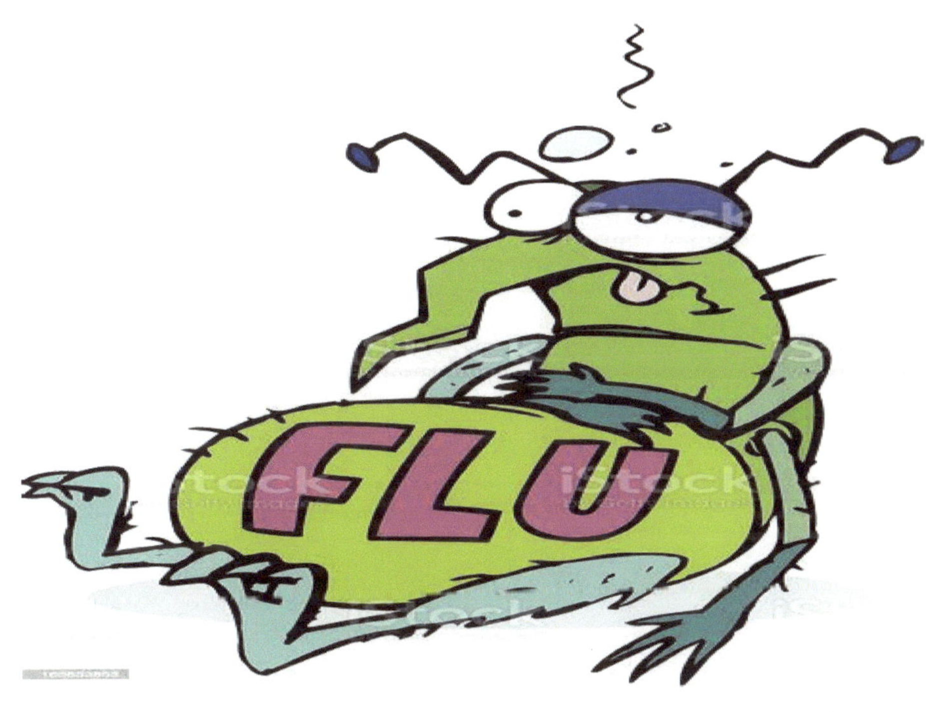

IT IS MUCH MORE

DANGEROUS THAN THE FLU

IT IS MUCH MORE CONTAGIOUS THAN THE FLU…

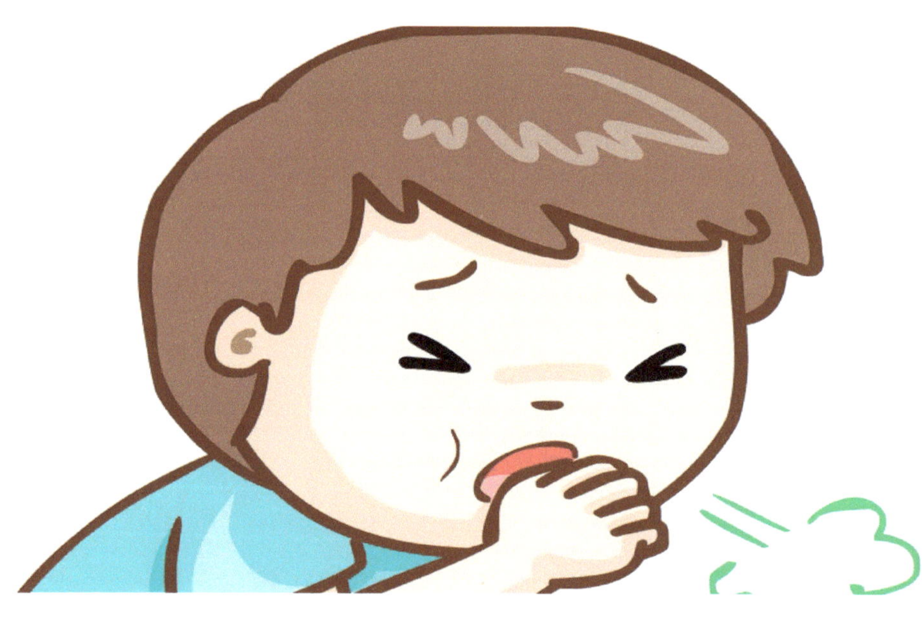

IT SPREADS FASTER THAN THE FLU

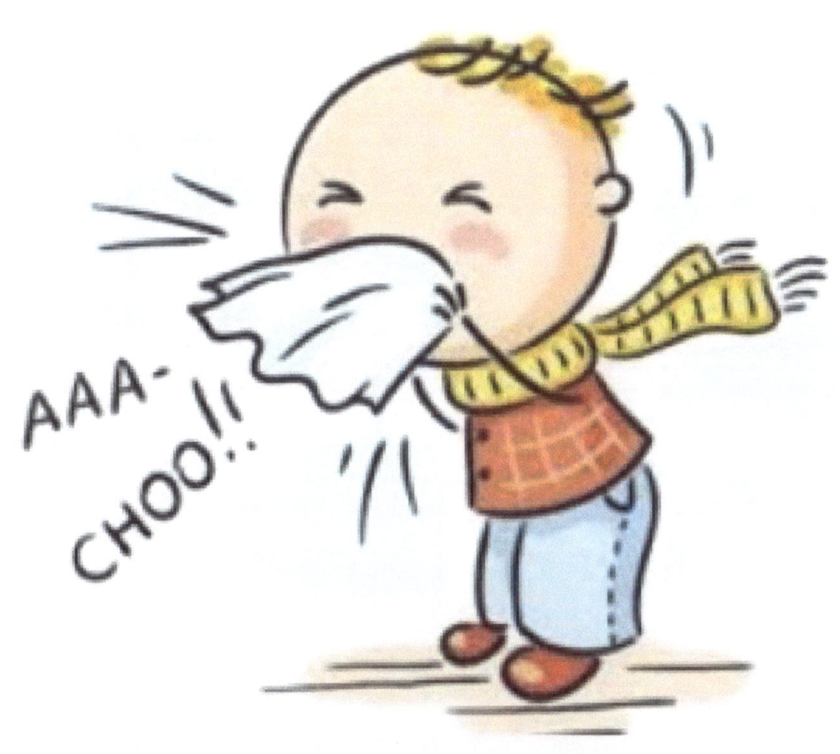

Chapter 2

SOME SYMPTOMS OF

COVID 19 INCLUDE :

FEVER OR CHILLS

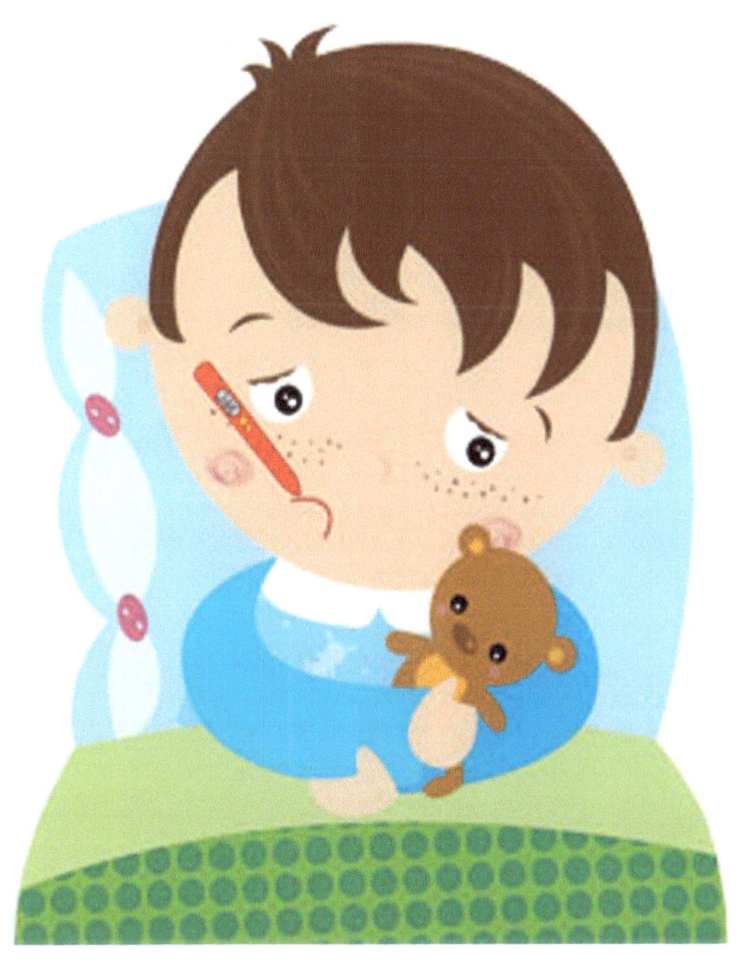

A REALLY BAD COUGH

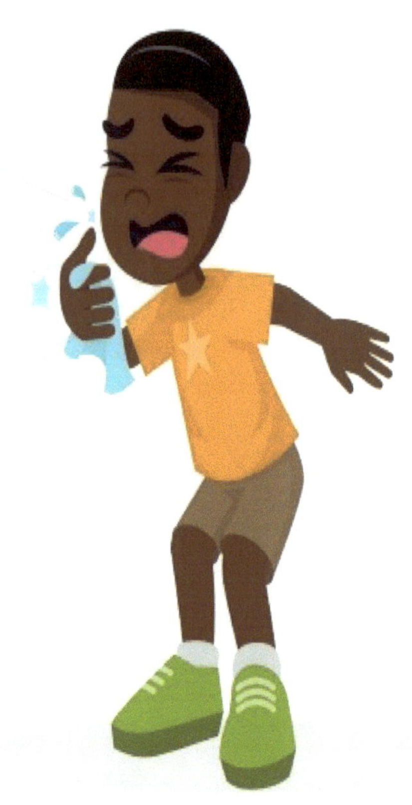

SHORTNESS OF BREATH

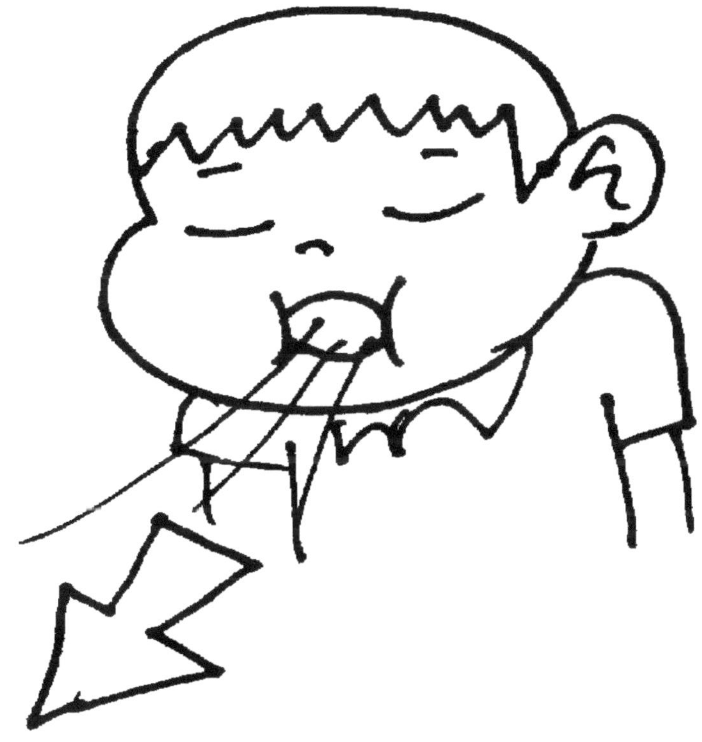

OR DIFFICULTY BREATHING

FATIGUE – EASY TO GET TIRED

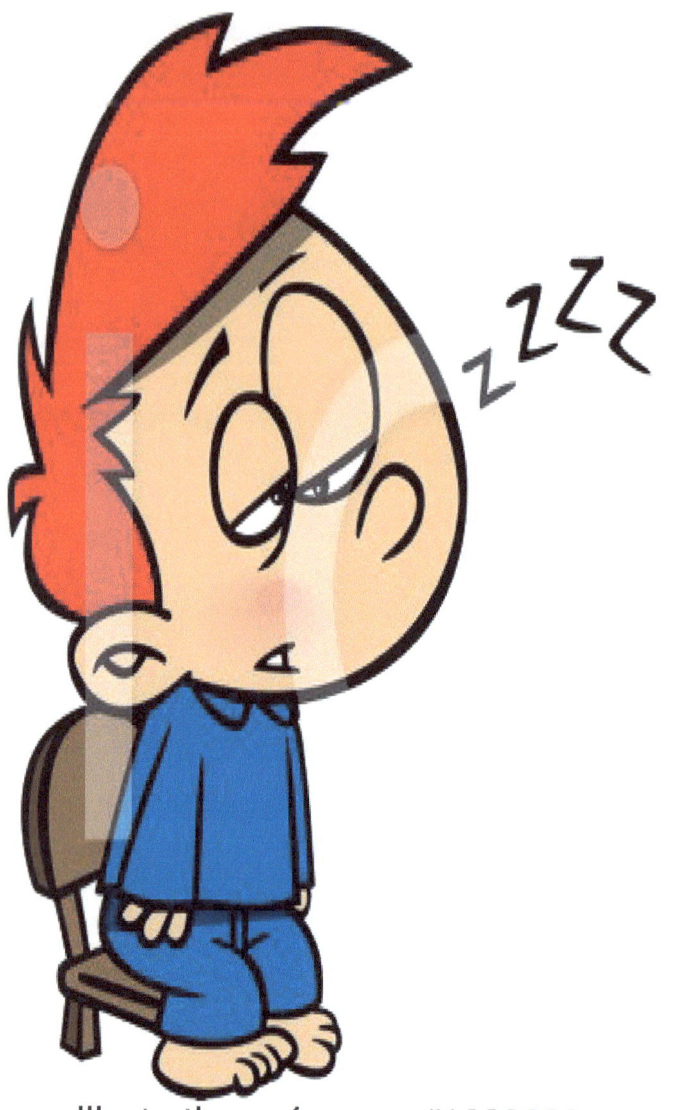

MUSCLE OR BODY ACHES

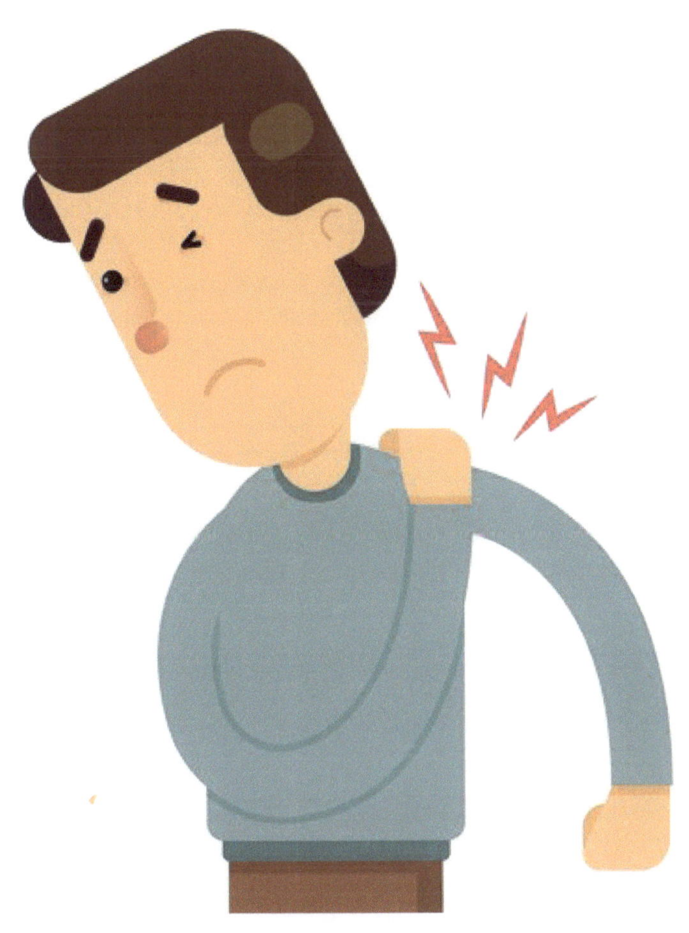

HEADACHE

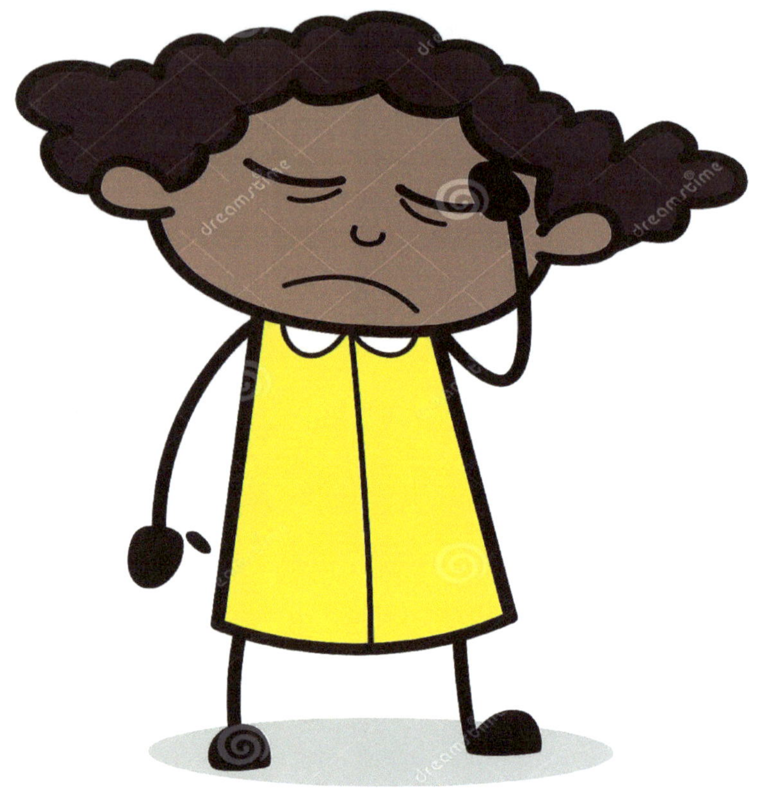

LOSS OF TASTE OR SMELL

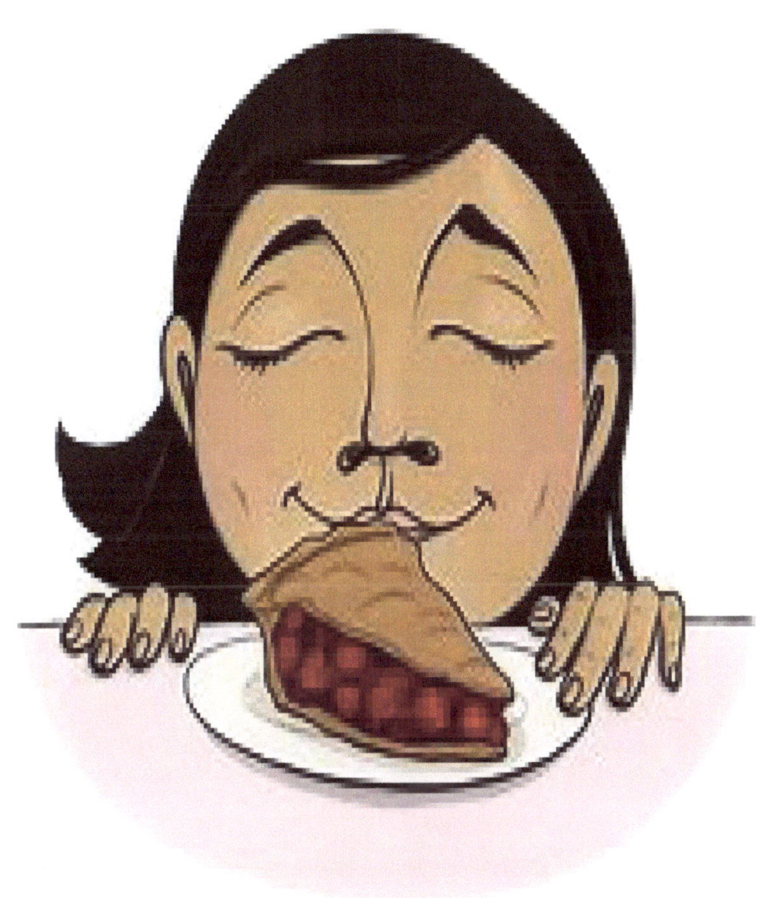

SORE THROAT

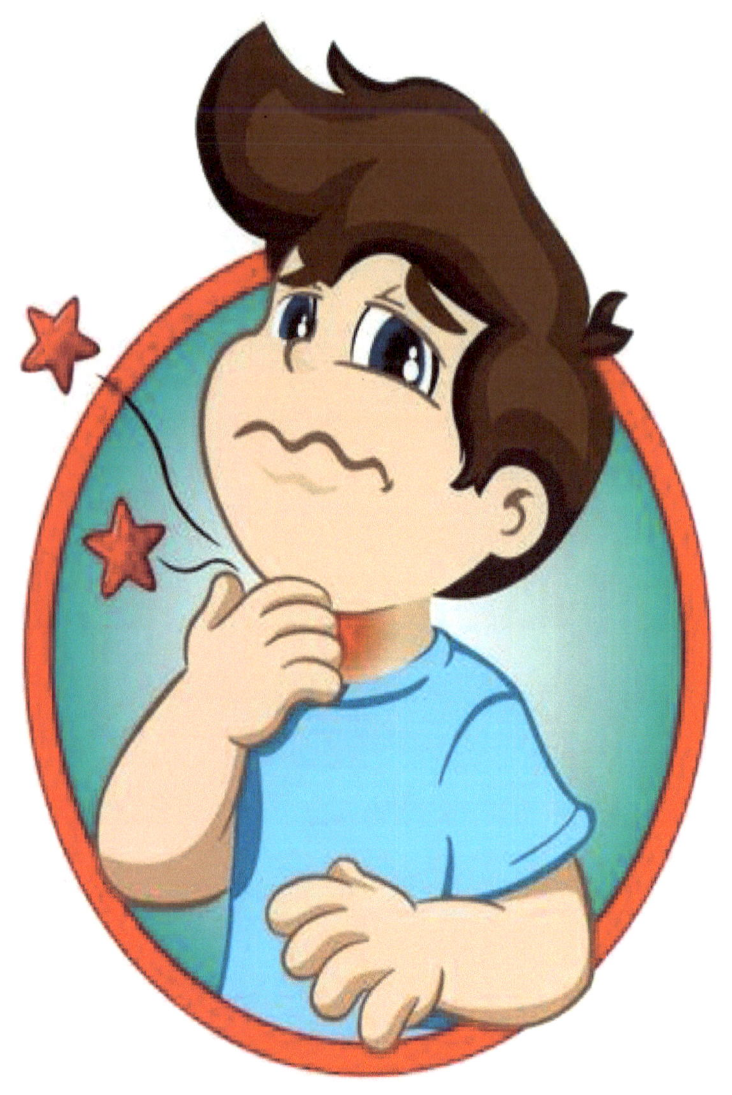

CONGESTION OR RUNNY NOSE

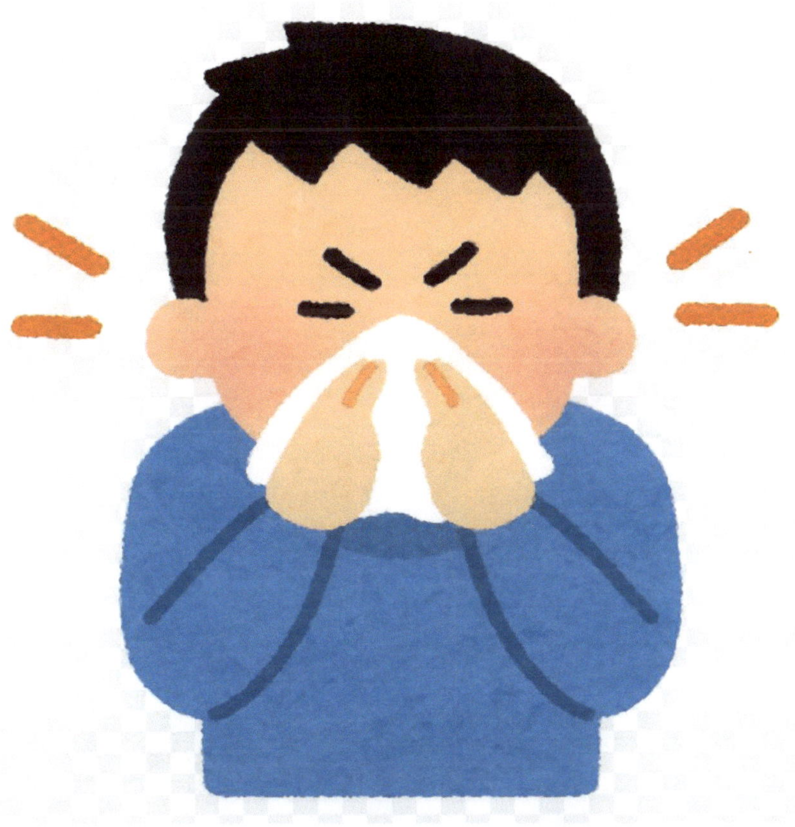

NAUSEA OR VOMITING

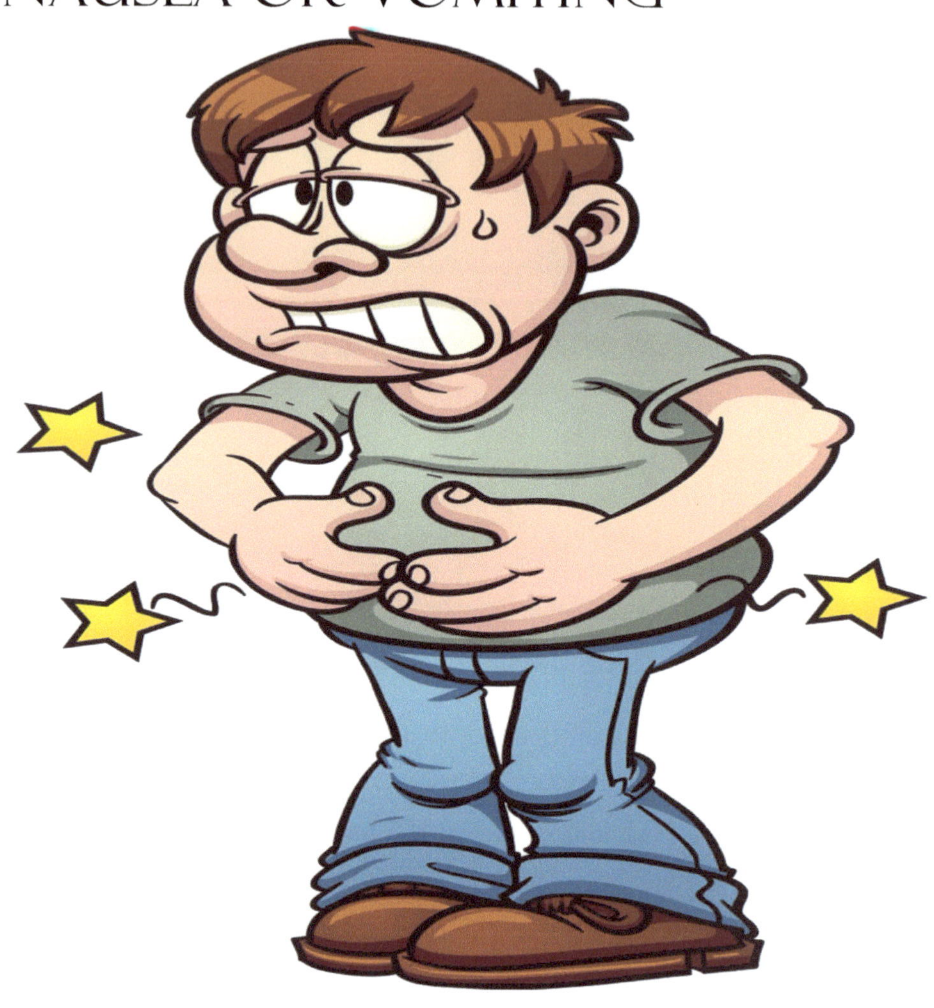

DIARRHEA

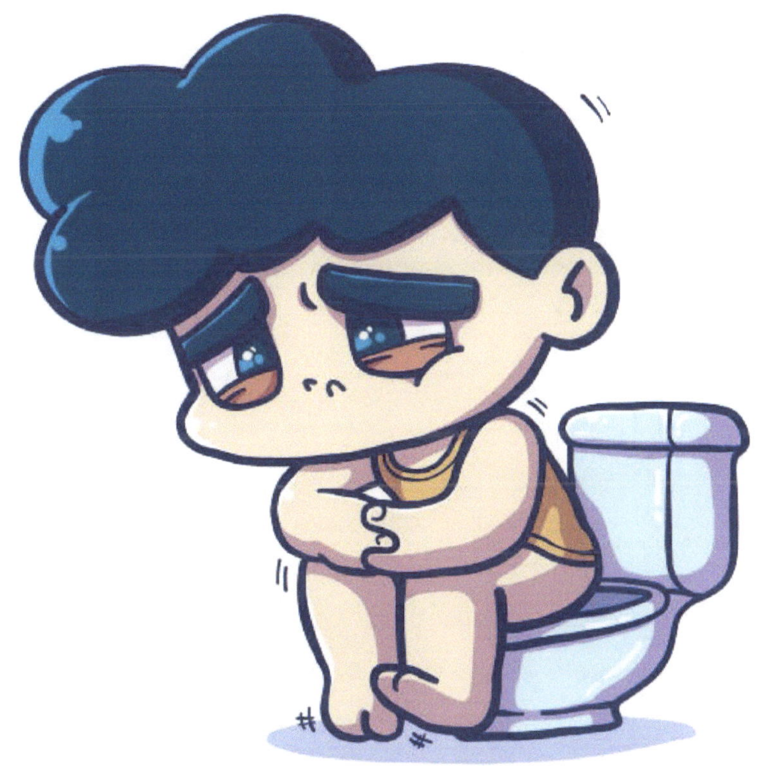

REMEMBER, THIS VIRUS CAN ONLY MAKE MORE OF ITSELF BY ENTERING LIVING CELLS (GERMS).

IT IS IMPORTANT NOT GETTING INFECTED

AND EVEN MORE IMPORTANT, NOT TO INFECT OTHERS…

TO DO THIS…

ALWAYS REMEMBER THE BIG

3 W'S

1.

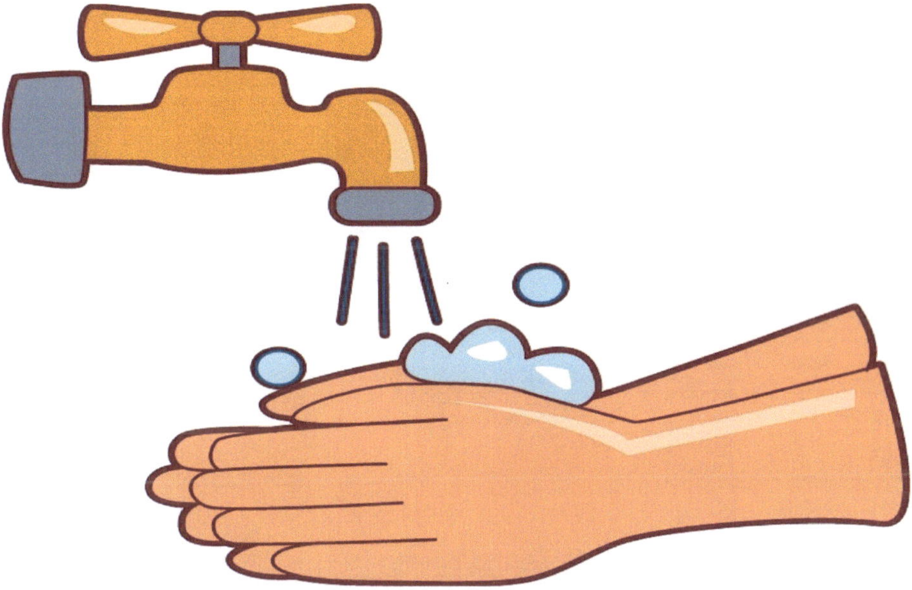

WASH YOUR HANDS........FOR
20 SECONDS OR MORE...

_{2.} WATCH YOUR DISTANCE….

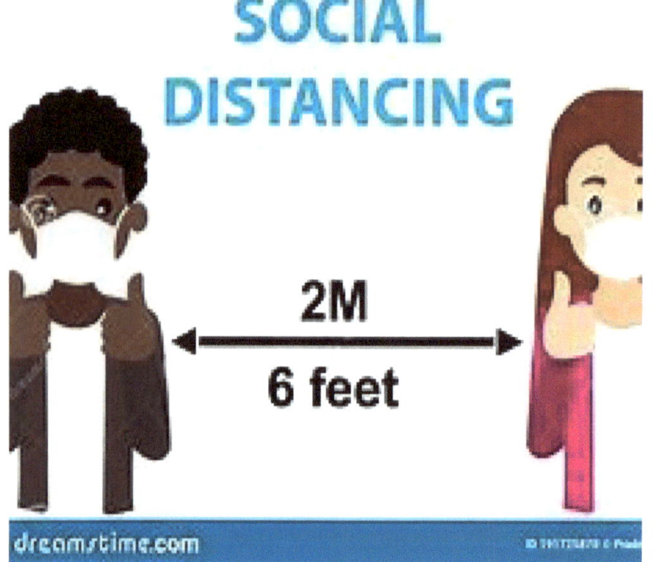

SOCIAL DISTANCING 6 FEET

WHEN YOU CAN

…..THIS MEANS "NO HUGGING," AND "NO HANDSHAKING"

3. WEAR YOUR MASK...

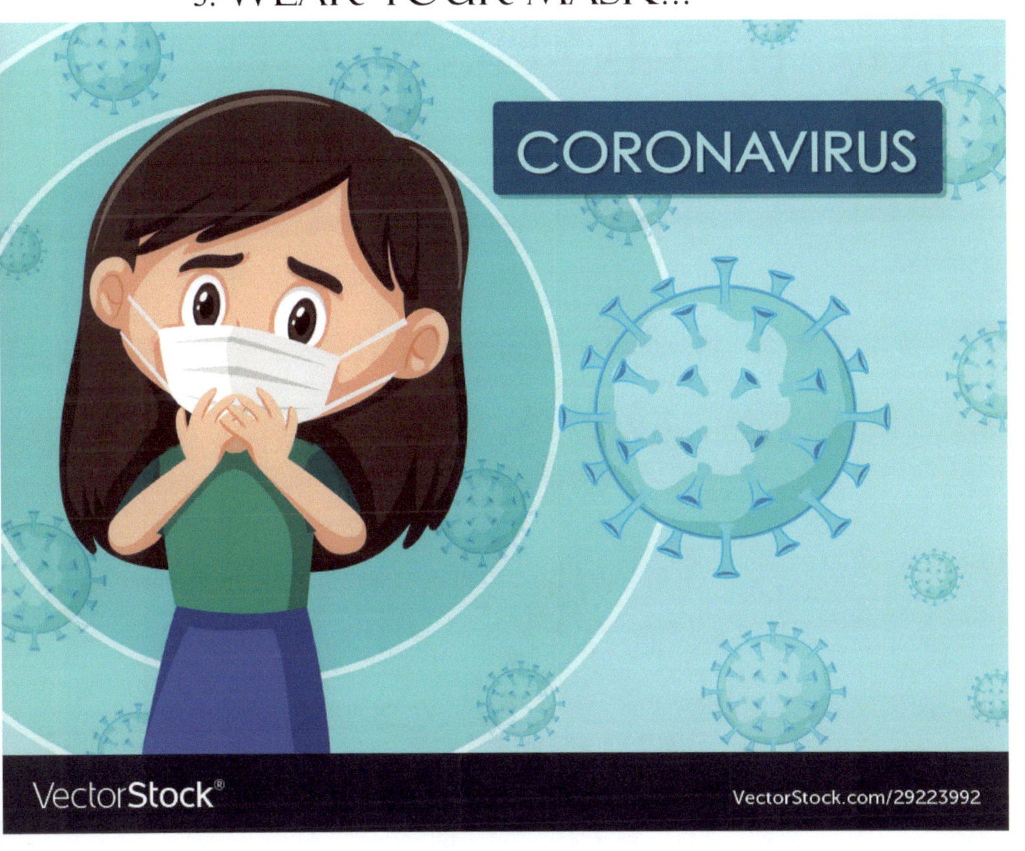

KN–95 MASK IS THE BEST!!!

4. STAY AT HOME WHEN AND IF DIRECTED TO PROTECT YOURSELF

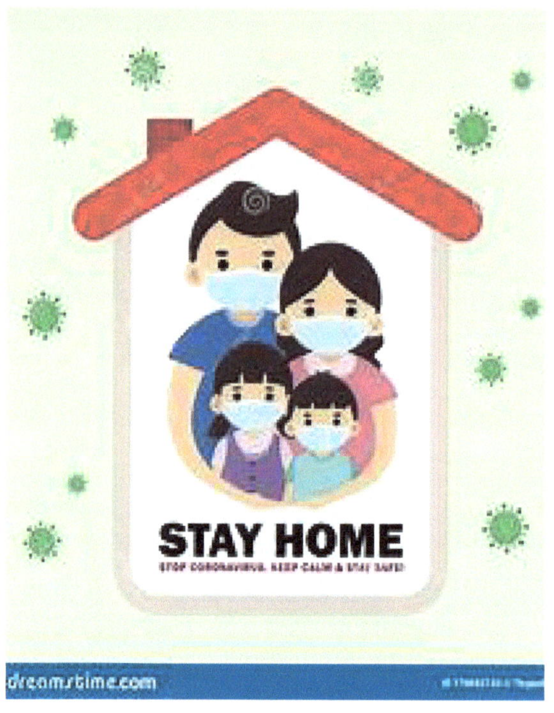

AND TO PROTECT OTHERS!

5. QUARANTINE IF AND WHEN DIRECTED BY AUTHORITIES

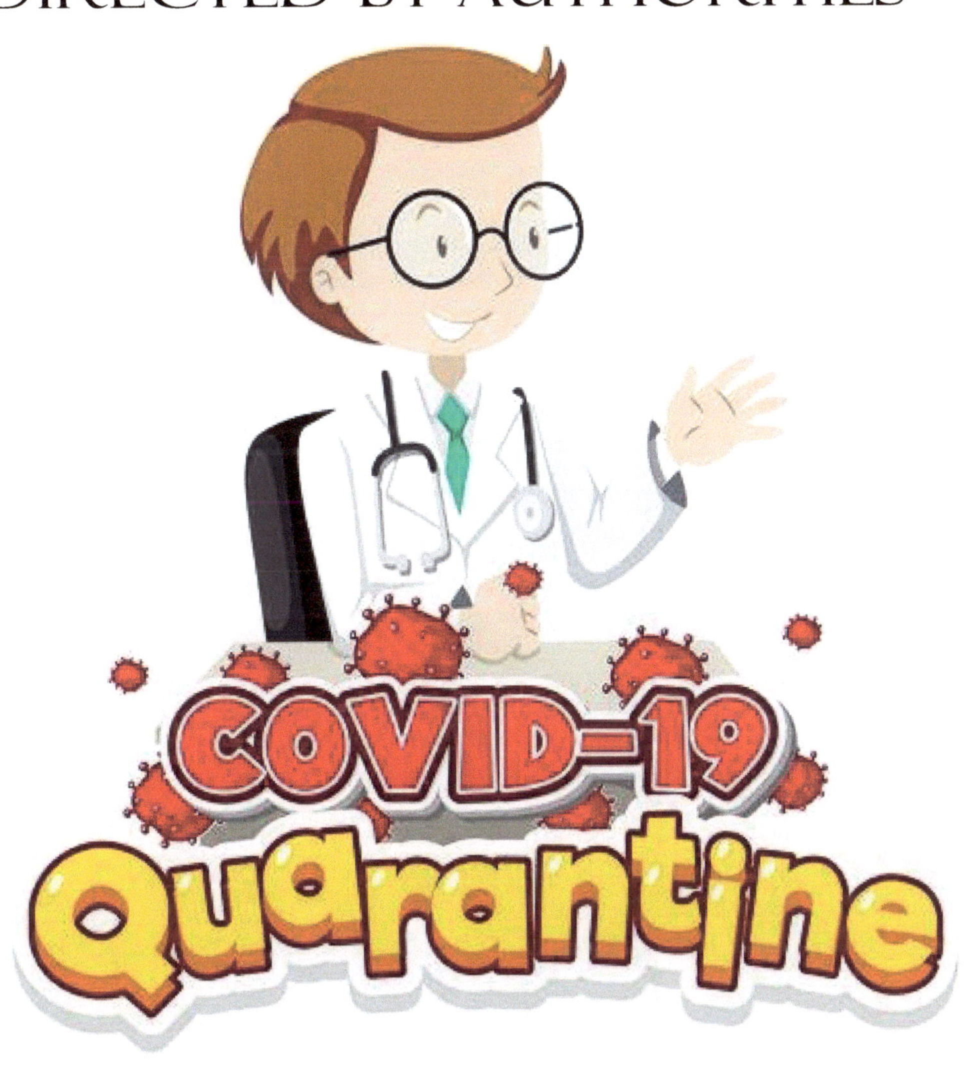

Chapter 3

LOGICAL NEXT STEP

WE ALL NEED TO COOPERATE WITH

THE SCIENTISTS WHO KEEP

US INFORMED…

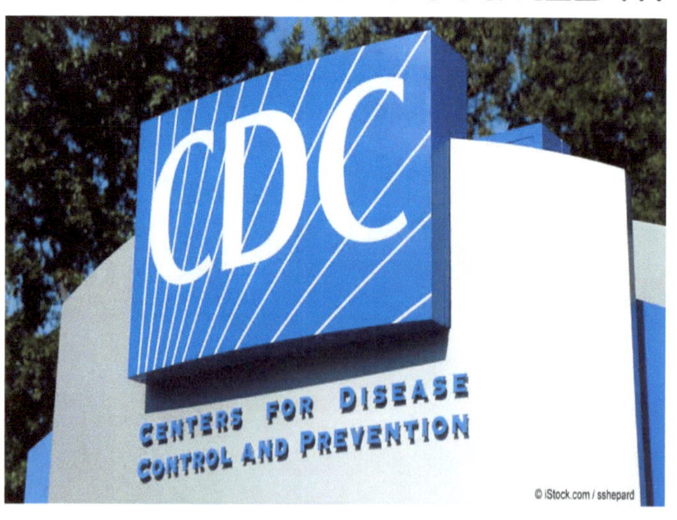

REMEMBER THE BIG 3 W'S

1. CONTINUE WASHING YOUR HANDS

2. CONTINUE WATCHING YOUR DISTANCE

3. CONTINUE WEARING YOUR MASK

GET VACCINATED AS SOON AS YOU ARE ELIGIBLE!

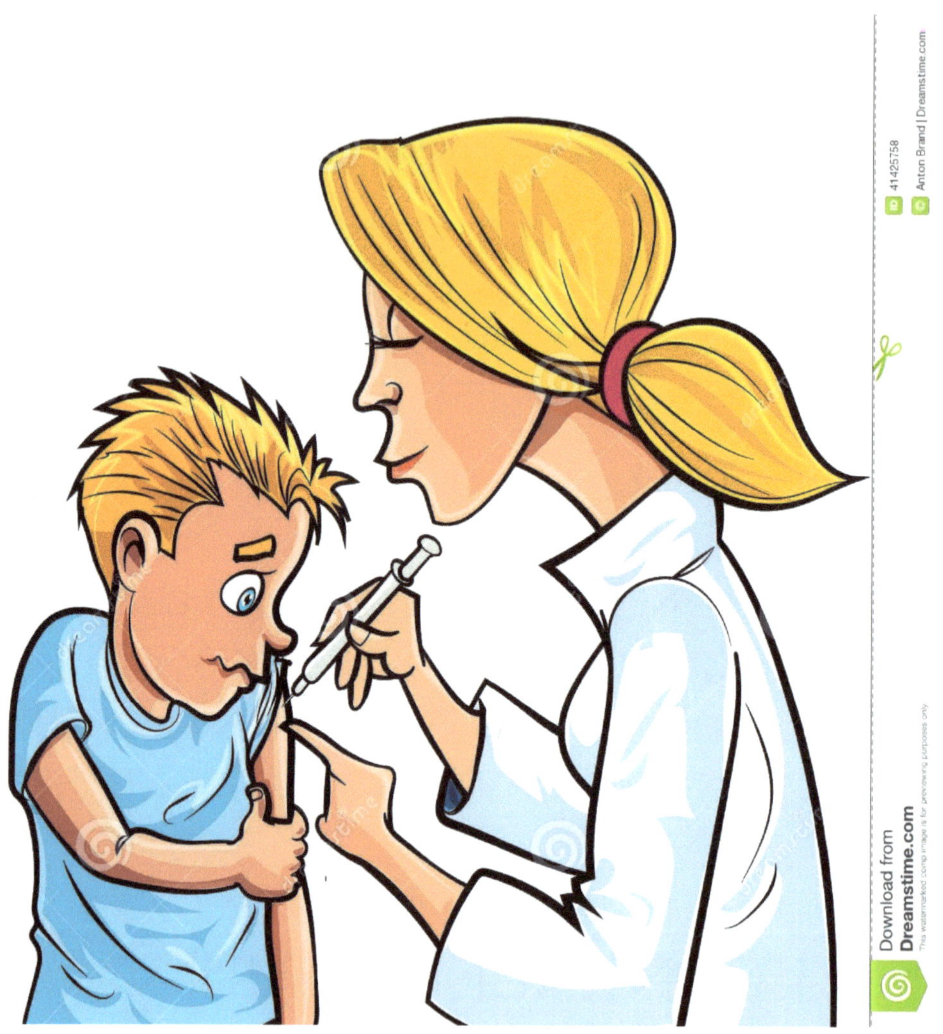

Chapter 4

Activity

DO YOU REMEMBER?

BEFORE COVID 19 BECAME A

MAJOR WORLD ISSUE, EVERYONE

WENT ABOUT THEIR BUSINESS

WITHOUT THINKING ABOUT

PERSONAL SAFETY OF OTHERS.

1. WE CRAMMED SPORTS ARENAS

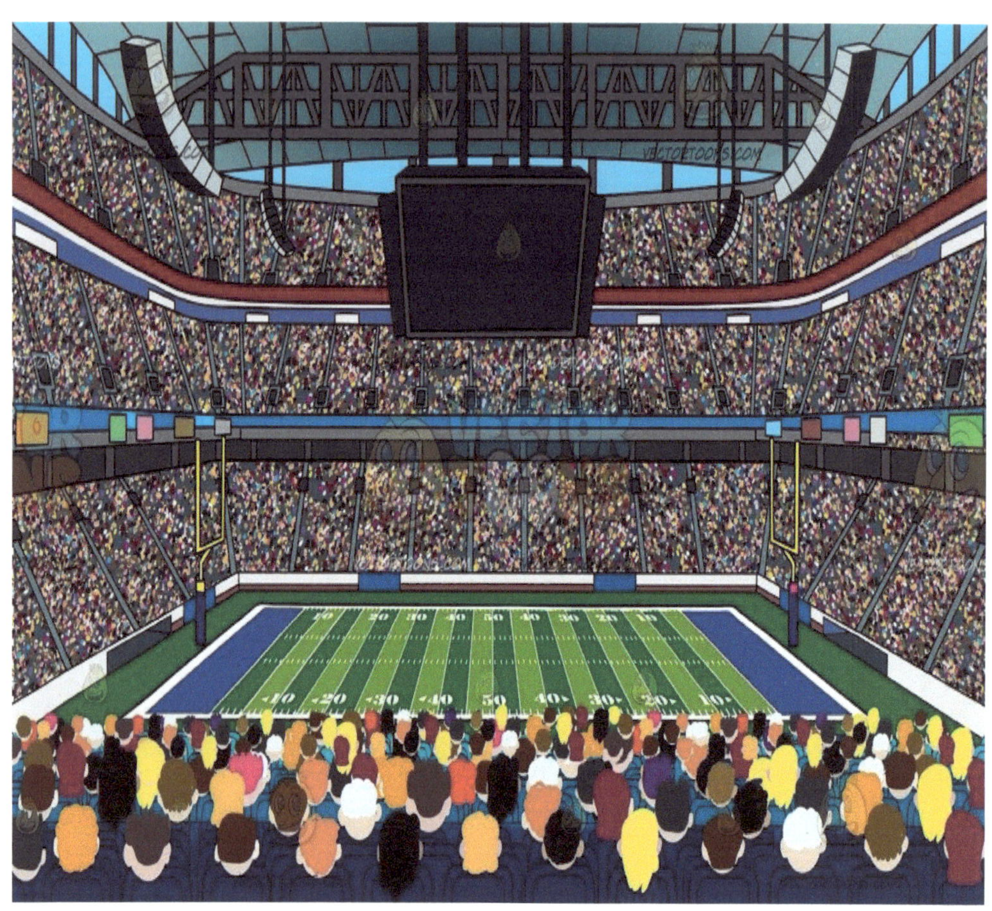

2. WE PACKED TOY STORES

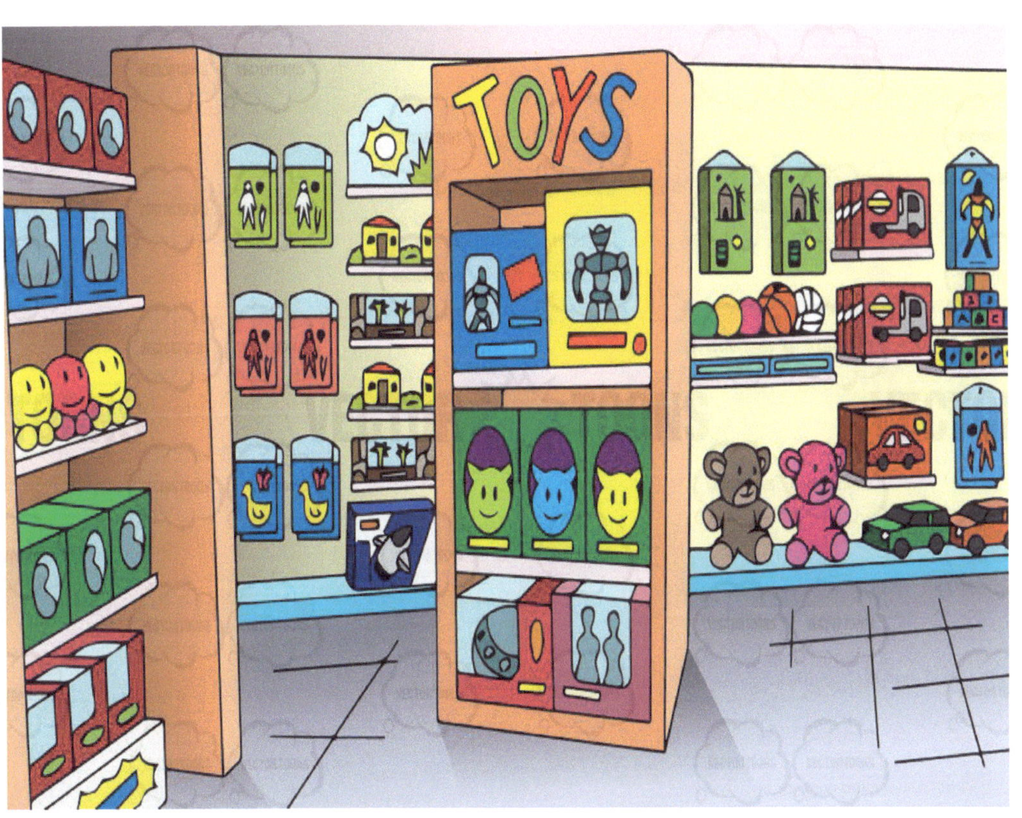

3. WE CONGESTED SHOPPING MALLS

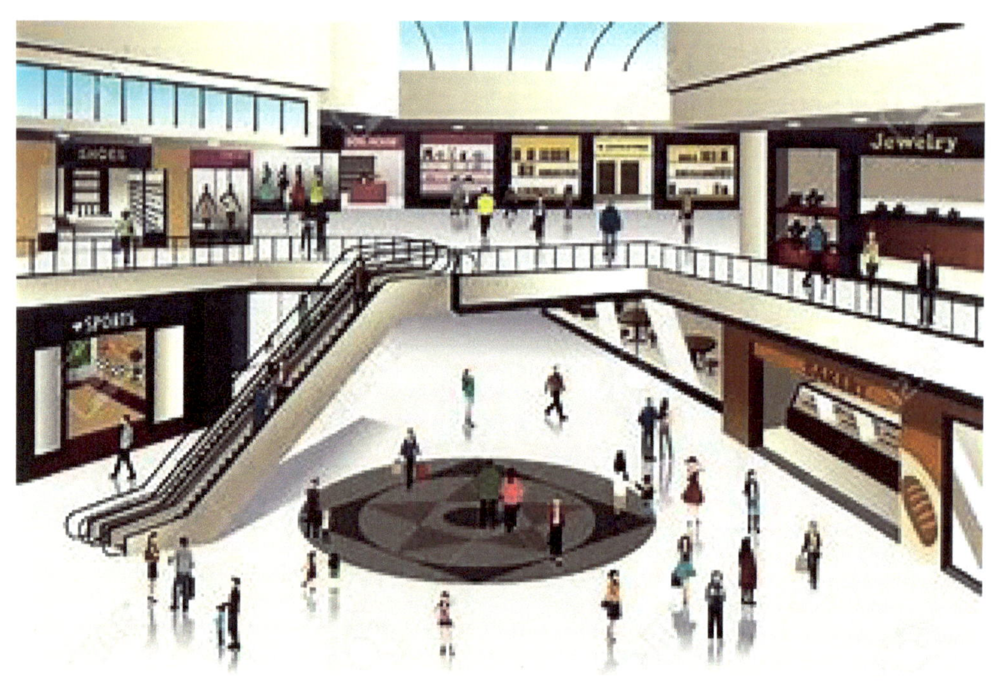

4. WE JAMMED GAMESTOP

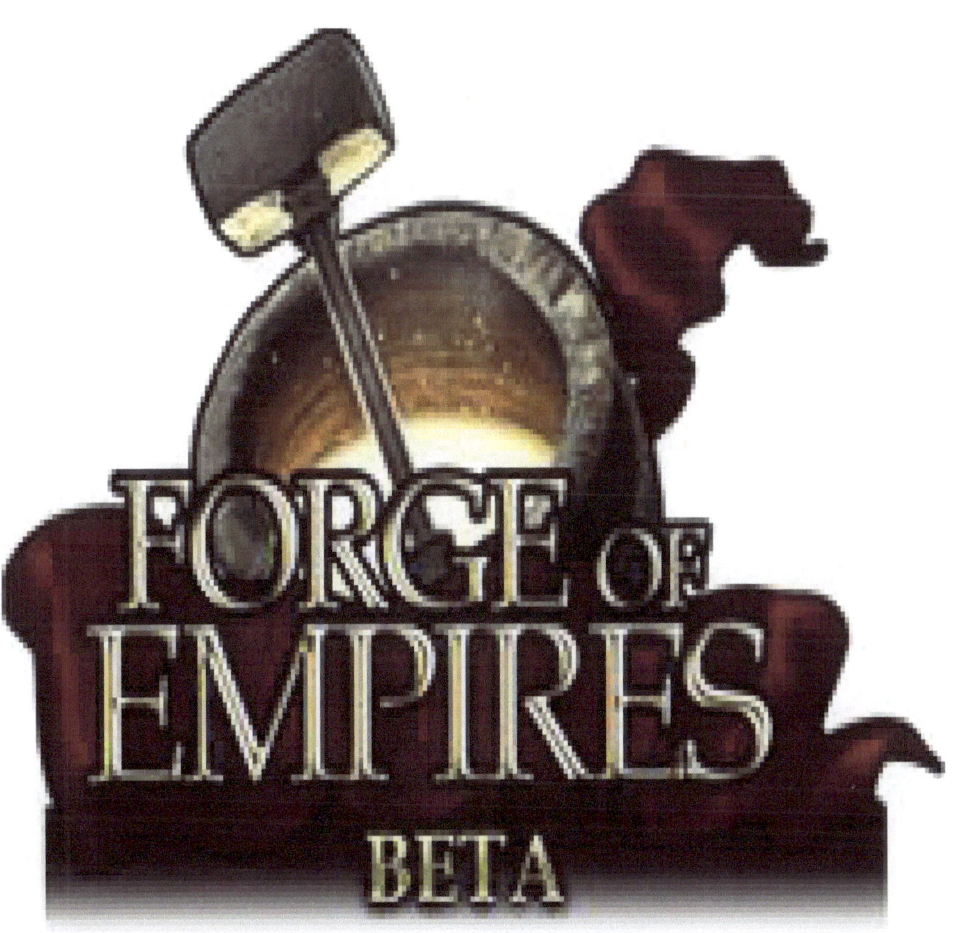

5. WE PACKED MOVIE THEATERS

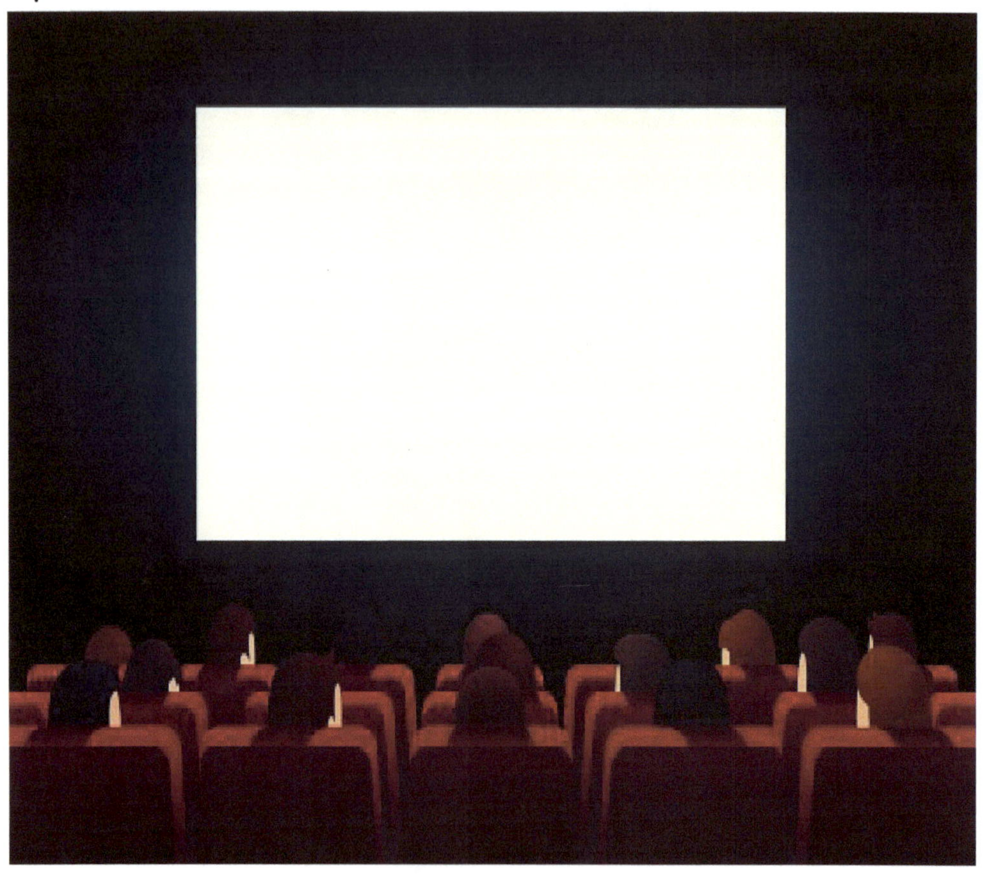

6. WE STORMED GROCERY STORES

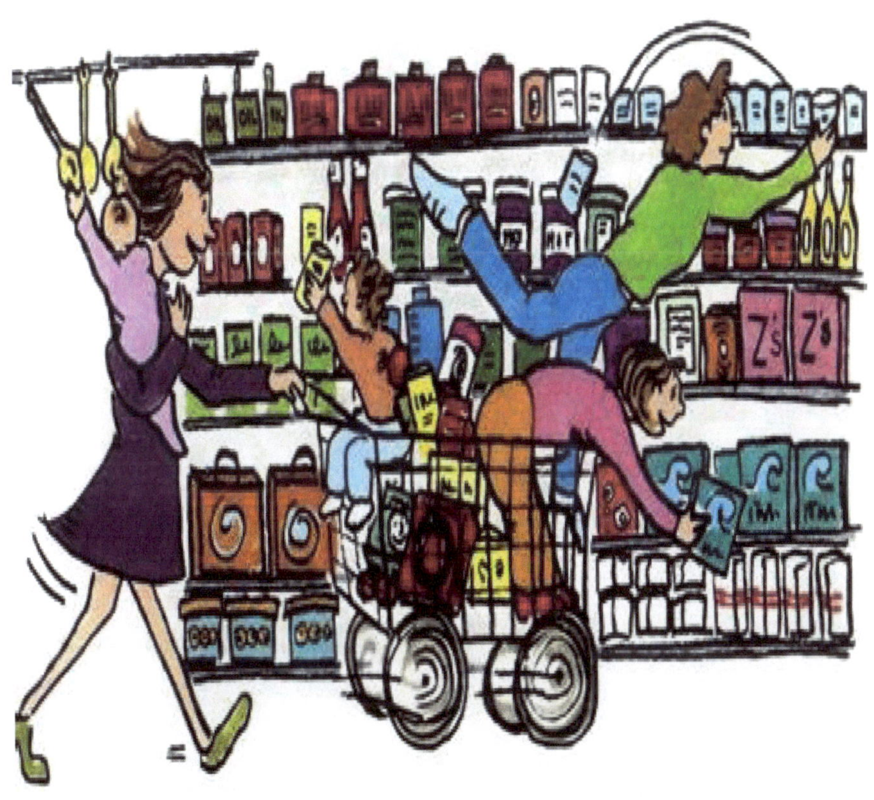

7. WE FILLED OUR CHURCHES

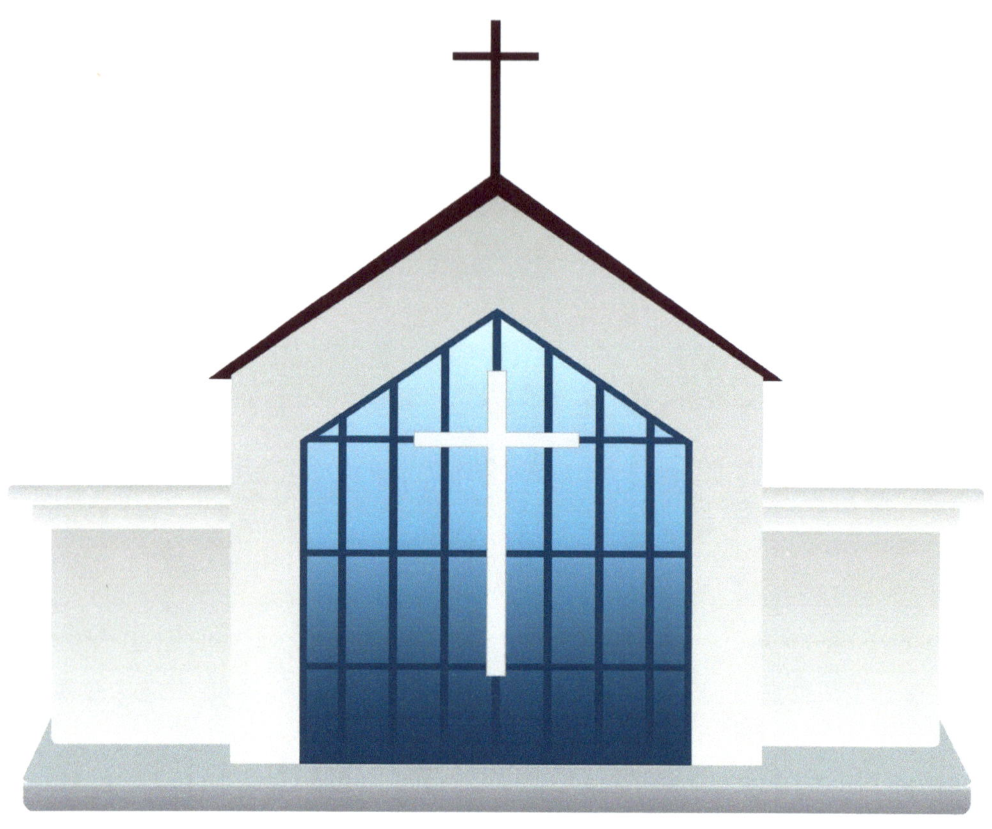

Accountability

OUR FUTURE IS UP TO US TO
PROTECT

OUR SAFETY IS UP TO US TO
PROTECT

CONTINUE TO WASH YOUR
HANDS

CONTINUE TO WATCH YOUR

DISTANCE

CONTINUE TO WEAR YOUR MASK

Chapter 6

The Future is Ours

ON THE POSITIVE SIDE, THE PANDEMIC'S CONDITIONS HAVE PRESENTED NEW OPPORTUNITIES FOR SELF-CARE FOR MANY PEOPLE — WITH <u>EXTRA TIME AT HOME</u> <u>FOR PROJECTS</u> SUCH AS PAINTING,

PLAYING MUSIC AND
EXPERIMENTING WITH COOKING
AND BAKING, MORE QUALITY
TIME WITH PETS, ADDITIONAL
EMOTIONAL SPACE TO JOURNAL
AND A RENEWED PREMIUM ON
DAILY WALKS.

Some Things My Friends Should Know about Covid-19

About the Author

My name is Dr. Anthony T. Craft, and I am a retired veteran Law Enforcement Officer of twenty-five years. I am also a retired Master Sergeant (E-8) from the United States Army Reserves, after serving twenty-eight years.

I earned my Ph.D. in Philosophy with a specialization in General Psychology from Northcentral University, September of 2021. I have earned two master's Degrees, the first in Rehabilitation Counseling from South Carolina State University in Orangeburg, SC., and the second in Criminal Justice from Florida Metropolitan University in Tampa, FL. I have taught Criminal Justice classes in a college environment, which I thoroughly enjoyed. I have one daughter,

Janika Shekelia Craft and two grandchildren, Devon and Daysha Grandberry. My goal is to provide helpful and exciting reading material to the public in the form of books, to assist our future investment in our children by educating them about what is happening around them every day.

Anthony presently resides in Irmo, SC.

Some Things my Friends Should Know about Covid-19

Advertisements

If you enjoyed my very first children's book, <u>Some Things my Friends Should Know about Covid-19</u>, please do not stop there. I have written two other books that I hope you will purchase and enjoy!

First Book:
<u>How to Conduct a Basic Crime Scene Investigation</u>
http://www.lulu.com/content/paperback-book/howtoconduct-a-basic-crime-scene-investigation/7641329

Second Book:
<u>Criminal Investigations –an- Officer's Perspective</u>
http://www.lulu.com/content/paperbackbook/criminalinvestigations-an-officersperspective/7872455

References

Centers for Disease Control and Prevention (CDC), "5.5 million visits to emergency departments in 2016 involved mental illness as the primary diagnosis" (2016, p. 24).

Kramer, J. (2021). Here's what the WHO Report found on the origins of Covid 19. National Geographic.

Magness, P.W., & Earle, p.c. (2021). The Origins of Political Persistence of Covid – 19 Lockdowns. *Independent Review, 25*(4), 503-520.

Pavlovic, N., Krstic, M., & Lakicevic, M. (2021). Performing the Activities of Travel Agencies in Serbia during Covid 19 Virus Pandemic. *Megatrend Review, 18* (1), 159-176. https://doi.org/10.5937/MegRev2101159P.

56